Why the Red Face: Dealing with Rosacea 101

By Chloe Hill

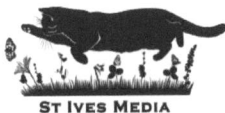

ST IVES MEDIA

First published in Australia in 2016
By St Ives Media
stivesmedia.com.au

St Ives Media
P.O. Box 52
Nunawading VIC 3131,
Australia

National Library of Australia Cataloguing-in-Publication data: (pending)

Hill, Chloe
        Why the red face: dealing with rosacea 101 / Chloe Hill
        ISBN: 978-0-99226757-5 (paperback)
        Acne
        Rosacea
        Acne Rosacea - Therapy
        St Ives Media
616.53

Cover design by: St Ives Media
Internal design by: St Ives Media

For Alan, as always

Contents

Introduction

This book is about the condition called rosacea.

If you're suffering from rosacea you'll have some or all of the following symptoms on your face or neck:

- Frequent blushing
- Facial redness
- Bumps (papules) and/or pimples (pustules)
- Sensitive skin
- Burning sensations and a hot feeling to the face
- Dry skin

You may experience these symptoms on a permanent basis or they may be 'triggered' by exposure to any of the following:

- Entering a warm building after being outside in cold temperatures
- Showering
- Exercise
- Socially stressful situations (such as public speaking or being the center of attention)
- Meals or alcohol
- Cosmetics or toiletries

You may also be about 40 years of age and someone who has blushed easily for most of your life, to the extent that people label you as shy or easily flustered.

If any or all of these conditions apply, you almost certainly have rosacea.

Naming your condition: Rosacea – what is it?

Rosacea (pronounced ROW-SAY-SHE-AH) n.

Is a chronic dermatitis of the face, especially the nose and cheeks, caused by the dilation of capillaries and is characterised by a red or rosy colouration acne like pimple. Also called *acne rosacea*.
[New Latin (acne) rosācea, *rose-coloured (acne)*, from Latin, feminine of rosāceus, *made of roses*;][i]

An important first step in dealing with any physical ailment is to get the correct name and diagnosis for your condition. Once your collection of symptoms has a name, you're considerably more progressed in seeking treatment and finding other like-minded people with similar symptoms to support you.

One of the big challenges for dealing with rosacea is also awareness.

Most people have never heard of rosacea and those who have generally have only a passing understanding of what it is. If they know more it's because a close friend or family member has the condition.

A recent survey done in conjunction with the National Rosacea Society of America and Galderma Laboratories revealed that just over half of rosacea sufferers either don't realise they have the condition or were not aware of treatments. They spent most of their energy trying to cover up the symptoms, not dealing with them. [ii]

Who should read this book

This book is aimed at people who are relatively new to an understanding of rosacea. It's been written to assist you to gain control over the problem for yourself and to help demystify what is happening to your body.

You may be newly diagnosed or have symptoms you're trying to understand. If you're like most people, in the early stages, you may be feeling overwhelmed by what is happening and at a loss to understand the patterns to your flare ups or to know if you can even do anything about them.

However you've come across this book - Welcome!

Not a trivial thing

Depending on your circumstance, your collection of rosacea symptoms can seem trivial or not even a condition at all. However the impacts to your social confidence can be devastating and it's important to minimise the effect it has on your life. Large numbers of people have an issue with rosacea every day and an estimated 45 million people worldwide are sufferers.[iii] While not exactly life threatening, rosacea is very real - don't let other people trivialise it.

Unfortunately, there's not a lot of seriously funded research into rosacea. Much of the management of the condition comes down to lifestyle changes and supplements rather than prescription drugs. Pharmaceutical companies simply don't have big enough incentives to fund research. It's not in the same league as a drug cure for cancer.

Some good news

The good news is that rosacea can be managed to the point where the impacts on your life can be minimal.

Regardless of your age, the natural healing systems in your body will do their work once you have recognised the condition and started to avoid or moderate exposure to your particular triggers. When you get your rosacea calmed down sufficiently you can allow the odd lapse in what you eat and put on your body and the effects will be marginal (if there are any at all).

As you review and eliminate trigger chemicals and foodstuffs you'll experience an improvement to your health in other ways.

Once you gain a sense of control over your symptoms you will feel reborn :-). You'll no longer be anxious about new experiences and environments that may lead to an embarrassing red face.

Every time you look in the mirror, you'll experience the satisfaction of seeing direct feedback that your efforts are making a difference, because improvements to your rosacea symptoms will be obvious to you.

My approach

I'm not a medical person; I'm a fellow rosacea sufferer. I've had considerable experience dealing with rosacea since I was first diagnosed about 15 years ago. I've researched the subject, talked to doctors and experimented with what works and what doesn't. My rosacea is now well under control and is something I rarely think about these days. In fact I've thought more about it since I began writing this book than I have in years.

I felt there was value in sharing what I've learned by putting together the sort of book that would have helped me in the beginning when I was first diagnosed and trying to make sense of it all.

There's a lot of information online about rosacea and it can be daunting to know where to start.

What I've tried to do is lay out some facts and areas of your life to consider then provide you with a plan to tackle your condition. For some of these areas, I've just scratched the surface to raise your awareness, you can pursue them more fully yourself later. I'm conscious this is a book about rosacea not a general health text.

Rosacea is a lifelong condition so consider this learning as an investment in you.

You can be confident this book is not an underhanded way of selling you anything or to hook you into a line of thinking. I'm an independent person with no affiliation to a product, organisation or service who is just trying to help you navigate your way.

New products are coming onto the market every day. Rather than be too prescriptive and give you a list of products, I've laid out some broad principles to guide you with making your own choices based on what's available to you locally.

I'd like to see you reach a point where you understand your triggers and your rosacea is under control. Any changes you've made are incorporated simply into your daily routines and you've stopped pre-occupying yourself with rosacea and got on with all the other worthwhile things in your life.

Chapter 1 - Rosacea Facts

Rosacea is a vascular disorder that affects an estimated 45 million sufferers worldwide. [iv] The condition is very common in people with fair skin who originated from England, Ireland and Northern Europe. A National Rosacea Society survey of 600 rosacea patients found 52% reported another family member who also suffered from rosacea and 42% indicated they were of Irish, German or English ancestry. [v]

While some ethnic groups may be more prone to rosacea than others this is only a relative observation.

Some people exhibit a tendency towards rosacea from an early age, these people have a life long issue with frequent 'blushing'. As people approach 40, the condition starts to make itself known by an almost permanent redness to the face (particularly the cheeks and forehead), although symptoms can first appear within the ages of 30-50. [vi] The redness is seen mostly on the face but can appear also on the neck, ears, chest and shoulders. People who have rosacea also frequently have problems with varicose and spider veins on other parts of their body. [vii]

Women experience rosacea more often (2-3 times more frequently than men) [viii] but men who are sufferers tend to have a more severe condition. Despite common myths, drinking does not cause the condition, nor is it caused by exposure of the skin to sunlight. It's a genetic 'luck of the draw' exacerbated by certain lifestyle factors.

Rosacea is sometimes mistaken for, or co-exists with acne or dermatitis.

The different types of rosacea

There are four different types of rosacea, which can exist singly, together or even form a progression from one to the other if left untreated.

1 **Erythematotelangiectatic rosacea**: Affected areas are permanently red and individuals tend to flush and blush more easily. Small blood vessels may be visible and individuals may experience a burning sensation.

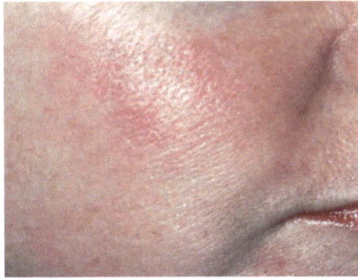

2 **Papulopustular rosacea**: Affected areas may be permanently red, with red bumps and whiteheads. This type is often confused with acne.

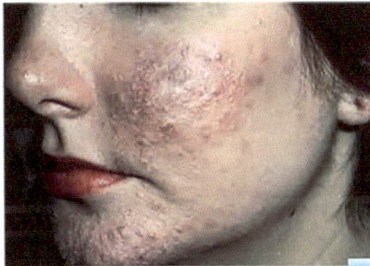

3 Phymatous rosacea: Affected areas are thickened, red, even bulbous, with enlarged pores and sometimes cystic acne or irregular surface nodularities. Small blood vessels may be visible. This type occurs more often in men (Bill Clinton, Boris Yeltsin and W.C. Fields are famous sufferers).

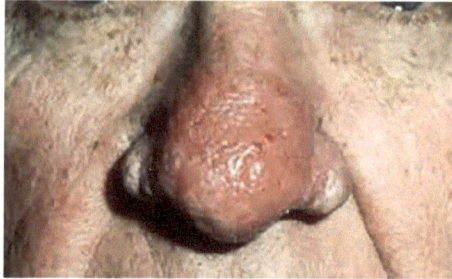

4   **Ocular rosacea**: Characterised by red, dry and irritated eyes and eyelids. Other symptoms include foreign body sensations, itching and burning.

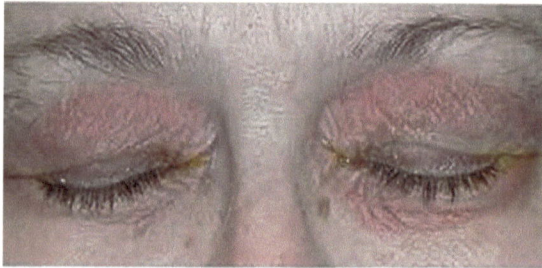

Some not so good news

You may come across books and websites which promote the complete eradication of rosacea, but such cures are a myth.

Certainly the condition can be moderated and contained to the point where it's no longer visible, but it will never be completely eradicated based on current advances in medicine. The honest truth is that you're stuck with rosacea lifelong.

Your body is not a machine and the triggers that lead to rosacea vary between people. Trying to understand the triggers that significantly affect you can be the most frustrating aspect of the condition. Unfortunately people who promote 'cures' and treatments can exploit this situation. Some products and supplements do wonders for certain people but for others are irrelevant. You can end up spending unnecessary money on trial and error.

You'll also come across books and websites offering false hope of a quick resolution for your rosacea. Getting this condition under control can take some months depending on your age and how severe your symptoms have become before you take action. You may have to be patient but improvements will be visible right away once you start recognising and minimising your triggers.

Becoming informed about rosacea via books like this is your best defense. This book will provide you with a sound basis on which to filter information about the condition and products that are presented to you. It will also prepare you to take on the role of educating friends, family and occasionally medical professionals about rosacea. Don't underestimate how stressful this can be on occasions.

Impacts of the "do nothing" approach

The "do nothing" approach to rosacea is not a good strategy in the long run because each time one of your triggers causes your face to redden unnecessarily the problem will only worsen. If left untreated the condition starts to appear almost permanently and is causing progressive damage to your system. Symptoms will only worsen without treatment and the situation can deteriorate quite quickly in as little as 6 months.

The appearance of rosacea indicates your body is out of balance. It's a wake up call to look at your health more holistically and to give the systems in your body the capacity to heal and work properly together. Think of it as a "canary in the coal mine" or an early warning that something is wrong and you have time to take some action.

The underlying cause of your symptoms

Rosacea appears on the outer layers of your skin but the problem originates in your vascular system and the deeper skin layers.

The body has a large number of natural processes, which occur daily to enable it to function. It's rather like a large metropolis or factory with many chemical reactions occurring.

One of these key processes involves keeping your body at its optimal temperature so the other systems can function most effectively. There are a large number of blood vessels and capillaries located around your face, which are in excess of what is required to transport nutrients to the area. These blood vessels appear to serve no other function than to assist with maintaining an optimal temperature for your all important brain to function. This excess of capillaries is however the seat of your rosacea symptoms.

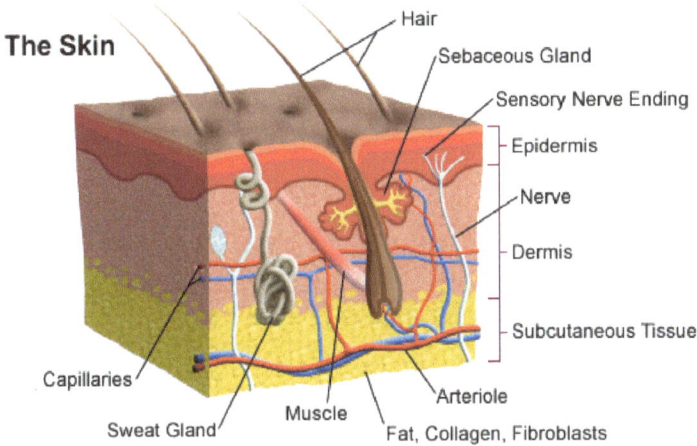

Diagram 1 - Skin structure

Diagram 1 - Skin structure shows the complex structure of the skin. The skin is the largest organ in the body and extremely dynamic. Dead cells in the outer layer are being removed and replaced by cells from the lower layers in a continuous cycle.

Your vascular system

The capillaries under the surface of the skin dilate when the external temperature is warm (or when you have been exerting yourself) and contract when the external temperature is cool. On a cold day the skin on your face is pale and your hands and feet get cool because blood is moving away from your body's extremities towards your core. By managing the heat exchange in this way you are able to keep your core body temperature at an optimal 37°C (98.6°F).

What happens with rosacea sufferers is that because there's an underlying weakness of the vascular system this leads to the body reacting to certain 'triggers' by excessive capillary dilation and flushing. The repeated expansion and contraction of these capillaries leads to them being expanded for longer periods until, in some cases, they are almost permanently enlarged and you have a red face all of the time. As the signs and symptoms appear to worsen, small blood vessels on the nose and cheeks may become visible through the skin as small red lines. This is called telangiectasia.

Decreasing your exposure to triggers will improve the appearance of your rosacea by reducing unnecessary instances of excessive flushing and redness to the face.

Your lymphatic system

The lymph system manages the fluid balance in the body and drains the excess away. The lymph system carries this excess fluid back to various lymph nodes located around the body. These nodes contain white blood cells that kill off infections. All lymph nodes are located in parts of the body close to arteries (armpits, groin and throat) which is why those parts of your body swell when you have an infection. The lymph system also has an important role to play in trapping and dealing with cancer cells in the body.

Due to the underlying weakness of your blood vessels some of this fluid spills over from your capillaries into the surrounding tissue. This overspill causes the other main rosacea symptom that is small white pustules. These look like pimples but are actually lymphatic fluid that has leaked out towards the surface of the skin. You know these pimple like bumps are caused by rosacea because they often appear and disappear very quickly, sometimes as rapidly as overnight. Unlike the usual sort of pimple that can be in evidence for a number of days. The skin may also feel warm and look puffy which is caused by irritation and fluid accumulating in the upper layer of the skin more quickly than the lymphatic system can drain it away.

Rosacea can cause progressive damage to your lymphatic system.[ix]

Your gut and digestion

There's also another strong body of evidence to suggest the appearance of rosacea is related to problems with your digestive system. Like your skin, your stomach and gut are another frontline defense system in direct contact with the outside world. The appearance of rosacea is said to indicate a low production of acids and enzymes in the gut that lead to poor food digestion and excessive bacteria.[x] Gut performance can be directly affected by lifestyle factors such as diet, state of mind and speed of eating.

From an owner or "user" perspective your stomach can be a neglected area. Many people, apart from knowing what types of food they like, don't usually think too much about what's happening when food hits their stomach, is digested and nutrients pass into their blood stream. It's natural not to think too seriously about your digestion until there's a problem because it's largely happening out of sight.

Any of the following stomach issues can indicate all is not well:

● Bloating
● Gas
● General pain
● Indigestion
● Constipation

Large numbers of chemicals responsible for your immune system are generated from your gastrointestinal tract, as are neurotransmitters such as serotonin that control your mood. No doubt that's the origin of the phrase 'comfort food' and why so many people take comfort in often eating too much of the 'wrong' kinds of food.

There are multiple benefits in getting this part of your body working more efficiently. A poorly functioning gut has been linked to a number of chronic health conditions[xi] as well as rosacea. What are sometimes thought of as factors to do with age are actually factors to do with lifestyle. Your body can take a lot of punishment, but less as you get older which may be another reason for the timing of rosacea with middle age.

Other related conditions

There are a number of other health conditions, which often appear alongside rosacea and are potential causes or exacerbating factors. Cause and effect can be difficult to prove conclusively but there are recurring patterns that seem to implicate both lifestyle and stress.

Menopause

Rosacea can occur during peri-menopause and menopause. The symptoms tend to reduce by the end of menopause.[xii] There is also evidence of a hormonal dimension to rosacea that explains why sufferers are predominately women.[xiii] 91% of sufferers can trace the first onset of their rosacea to a traumatic episode or a period of intense stress,[xiv] which could include pregnancy or menopause.

Suppressed immune system

The correlation between rosacea and a suppressed immune system links back to the role your gut plays in your overall health. A suppressed or compromised immune system is further indication of a problem with your overall stress response and diet. [xv]

Migraine disease and (other) vascular disorders

Migraine sufferers have a higher incidence of rosacea than the average population. This correlation appears due to the vascular nature of migraines that also involve abnormal expansion and constriction of blood vessels.[xvi]

Demodex mite

Demodex mites are one of the organisms living on our bodies near hair follicles. Normally they cause us no problem. There's no conclusive evidence linking Demodex mites to rosacea but their presence has been identified as the cause of some skin diseases. They may only become an issue when immune systems are compromised and people are under stress. Demodex mites are touched on here because they're frequently mentioned in the literature about rosacea.

In summary

There's no single obvious cause of rosacea, but interplay between the following factors seems to be at its core:

- Age
- Sex (hormones)
- Diet
- Genetic disposition
- Lifestyle
- Stress

Chapter 2 - Rosacea Triggers

Areas of your life to consider

In the previous sections we covered what is going on in your body to produce rosacea symptoms. In the next section we'll discuss some of the common triggers that lead to rosacea flare-ups.

The concept of triggers will become extremely familiar to you, and as mentioned previously, not all triggers apply to each person. The best approach to narrow down the ones that apply to you is to systematically maintain a diary. The diary will help you assess situations where you are exposed to a number of potential triggers simultaneously and make identification and elimination easier to target.

Triggers

Triggers for the rosacea flushing response typically fall into one or more of the following four categories:

- Environment
- Food/Drink
- Products/Chemicals applied to the skin
- Mind/Lifestyle.

Environment

Many rosacea sufferers have sensitive skin, which responds acutely to changes in air temperature.

The most common situation is when you enter a heated building after being outside in the cold air. Or you are inside a building but move into an overheated room with a lot of other people.

The following situations may also trigger flushing:

Outside weather conditions
Exposure to hot sun, strong winds, excessively cold, humid or dry air.

Physical exertion
Physical exertion (even when mild), exercise, manual jobs involving lifting, getting excited or having an animated conversation.

Exposure to heat sources
Hot showers, baths, saunas, kitchens, heaters, open fires, bedding etc.

What you can do

Protect your skin from the environment
- Moisturise well and wear sunscreen all year round. Stick with products that are closer to Sun Protection Factor 15 (SPF15) as the stronger products that are as high as SPF30 or 50 may be more irritating to your skin. A good sunscreen or moisturiser with SPF works as a barrier cream not only for sun but also for wind, warm temperatures and pollutants in the air.

- For women wear a light foundation every day (preferably one with a good SPF) which also provides barrier protection.

Transition from cold to hot
- Be conscious of situations where you move from cold to hot air, protect your skin as much as possible with a scarf, high collared clothing or hood so there is a light layer between your face and the outside temperature.

- Where possible moderate the contrast between extremes of temperature. If you are someone who walks quickly, try slowing down. Move slowly into a foyer and acclimatise yourself before you move further into the building.

Layered clothing

- Wear layered clothing so when you transition between temperatures you're able to cool your body down quickly. A frequent cause of a red face is that you are simply too warm. Wear the type of layered clothing you can strip off relatively quickly and still leave yourself decently or professionally dressed (if it's the workplace).

- Wear natural fibres or manmade fabrics that breathe.

- Be cautious with items of clothing like singlets and under garments as these can keep you very warm but, depending on the temperature, can be difficult to discard if you start to overheat. Save these types of clothes for really cold weather or when you are outside.

- Don't be tempted to severely underdress in an effort to manage your body heat and facial redness. It's not good for your health and reflects a mindset that it's acceptable to 'suffer' for your condition. Instead make smarter choices about the types of fabrics and layers you wear.

Control your environment as much as possible

- In environments you can control keep the temperature down. Heating set higher than about 20-21°C (68-69.8°F) is wasteful and will contribute greatly to your heating bills and to global warming.

- Use humidifiers or set up bowls of water to get more moisture into the air. Drier air leads to faster dehydration making you feel hotter.

- Avoid very hot showers, baths, saunas, swimming pools and spas.

- When outside temperatures are moderate stay out of artificial environments and get as much fresh air on your skin as possible. Artificial environments are dehydrating and play havoc with your skin. They also interfere with your body's natural ability to maintain its temperature and dry out your mucous membranes, affecting your immune system and contributing greatly to the higher incidence of winter colds and flu.

- Be conscious of your proximity to all sources of heat. For example, while cooking in the kitchen or consuming temperature hot food and drinks. This is where your layered approach to clothing will help you. At the **first sign** of feeling warm, take off a layer to allow your body to cool down as quickly as possible. Attacking the problem quickly is your best mechanism to reduce the potential for flushing - don't try to ignore the feeling of overheating.

- A quick way to cool down is to run cold water over your wrists. This technique is effective because here veins are close to the surface of the skin and your circulation will cool down the rest of your body.

- Consider changing your work environment, or any environment where you spend considerable amounts of time, to one where temperatures are not so artificially controlled. You may even want to move location to a more sympathetic climate. Easier said than done, but people move locations all the time and you may consider the benefits worth the effort.

Stay hydrated
- Drink plenty of water to both keep hydrated and to assist your body with regulating temperature.

Adjust your sleeping habits

- Pay attention to the arrangement of your bedding. You may find you are overheating at night and need to switch to lighter covering. Blankets rather than duvets or a lighter weight duvet. You certainly shouldn't be over heating, sweating or casting off bedclothes at night on a regular basis.

- One strategy you can use to help with overheating while in bed is to fold up the blanket or duvet at the very bottom corner of the bed near your feet. This will act like a venting system. Especially useful if you share a bed with someone and your bedding arrangement is not exclusively your own.

- At night you may also want to turn down the heating or even turn it off depending on the temperature to ensure a cooler and less drying environment for your sleep.

Food/Drink

A good rule of thumb when assessing food is to remember:

The more processed the foodstuff, the greater potential issue for your rosacea

Good advice generally!

The chemical levels of some processed foods can be excessive. This leads to a chemical imbalance where you consume high amounts of some chemicals in relation to others. This degree of imbalance interferes with the body's ability to process ALL foods and chemicals.

Changing the types of food you eat by eliminating some foods and monitoring the speed with which you eat your meals are achievable changes that will improve your rosacea and allow your body to heal.

Common food triggers

Below is a table of foods commonly recognised as rosacea triggers. Some of these foods you may eat regularly and others you may be unfamiliar with.

The table also highlights foods containing:

- Histamines** or chemicals known to trigger the release of histamines in the body.
- Nitrates/nitrites$
- Sulfites#

All of these chemicals have been identified as rosacea triggers. You may notice certain foods such as beer contain a number of them. These foodstuffs tend to be a common trigger for many people (Further information about the impact of these chemicals below).

Table 1 - Foods recognised as common rosacea triggers

(**Foods high in histamines or triggers to release histamines into the body, $foods high in nitrates/nitrites, #foods high in sulfites)

Fermented Alcoholic Beverages	Fermented Foods	Vinegar Containing Foods	Cured Meats
Red wine**#(Sulfites also occur in white wine)	Vinegar**#	Olives**	Bacon**$
Champagne**	Soy sauce**	Some canned vegetables	Salami**$
Beer**#	Yogurt**	**Most Citrus Fruits****	Pepperoni**$
Bourbon	**Dried Fruits#**	**Vegetables**	Luncheon meats**$
Vodka	Figs**	Avocados**	Hot dogs**$
Gin	Raisins**	Eggplant**	Ham$
Soured Foods	**Fresh Fruits**	Spinach**	**Aged Cheese**
Sour cream**	Red plums	Tomatoes**	Hard cheeses
Dairy Foods	Bananas	Artichokes	Mould based cheeses (such as Blue Vein)
Diet drinks	Papaya**	Broad leaf beans (including pods) such as lima or pea	**Temperature hot food and beverages**
Vanilla	Pineapple**	Yeast extract (supplement not in bread)	Liver
Desserts#	Strawberries**	**Fish****	**Crustaceans****
Nuts**	**Spicy Foods****	Liquorice**	Egg white**
Peanuts**#	Chocolate**	**Frozen vegetables#**	
Many artificial preservatives and colourings**			

This list can look daunting, particularly if you're in the habit of eating a conventional Western diet as there are a lot of commonly eaten foods in the table.

To break the categories down further here are a number of things to note:

Food manufacture and preparation

Differences between food manufacturers and preparation methods leads to variation in the amount of chemicals found in each of these foods; as do regional and brand differences. In some cases the chemicals are artificially added while in others they occur naturally in the foods themselves. This lack of standardisation leads to confusion and to a wider group of foods making the list. It also helps to explain why there is such variation in the triggers between people.

Fresh food

You will also notice naturally occurring and fresh foods such as fruits and vegetables. These are whole foods but may contain chemical triggers to a greater or lesser degree based on seasonable or regional variations. The extent to which these types of foods affect you may depend on your level of sensitivity and the number of flare-ups you're experiencing. The trigger impact of these more naturally occurring foods will be considerably reduced as you proceed with getting your condition under control

Food Storage

Storage methods and length of storage time are also a consideration. Chemicals such as histamines increase when food is old or has been stored for too long. This will occur in even fresh, unprocessed foods.

Histamines, Nitrates/Nitrites, Sulfites

As mentioned earlier, there's considerable overlap between foods high in histamines, nitrate/nitrites and sulfites and foods causing a problem for rosacea sufferers. All these chemicals occur both naturally and are added to foodstuffs in manufacture.

Histamine intolerance

The word histamine is generally found in the context of anti-histamine drugs so most people can be forgiven for not realising it's also a naturally occurring chemical created in the body. Histamine is a neurotransmitter affecting your nervous, digestion and immune systems as part of your allergic response. It's also a key component of your stomach acid, aids digestion and regulates sleep, blood pressure and brain function.

As a general rule, histamines are added to processed foods that are aged (think about any type of fermented food - cheese, canned foods, beer etc.). Histamines also develop in food that's spoiled and starting to go off. The chemical can accumulate in your system over time which is one of the reasons why, if the condition is left untreated, rosacea sufferers get into a very sensitive state where even the smallest amounts of a foodstuff can cause a flare up.

Women appear to be more susceptible to histamine intolerance because of interplay between estrogen and histamine.[xvii]

Diamine Oxidase (DAO)

Diamine Oxidase (DAO) is the main enzyme that metabolises histamine in the body and is found in the small intestine and the upper colon. Low levels of Diamine Oxidase are often implicated in histamine intolerance.

There following foods block DAO and lead to histamine build up in the body:

Table 2 - DAO Blocking Foods

Alcohol	Energy Drinks	Black Tea	Mate Tea
Green Tea			

Nitrates and Nitrites

Nitrates occur naturally in some fruits and vegetables and it's estimated that about 80% of the nitrates consumed in a diet are from plant-based sources.[xviii] [xix] Nitrates and nitrites are used interchangeably as preservatives and nitrates once consumed convert to nitrites in the body.

Nitrates have an important nutritional role to play in the health of the cardiovascular system and eaten as part of a whole food have been known to have a positive impact on the body by lowering the blood pressure.[xx] Conversely excessive consumption of nitrates leads to vascular problems such as rosacea.

The amount of nitrates used as a preservative in cured meats such as bacon, ham, Frankfurt's, hot dogs, salami etc. may be well in excess of average daily requirements.

Sulfites

Sufiltes are used as a preservative in foods such as beer, wine, fruit juices, dried fruits, desserts and frozen vegetables as well as occurring naturally in foods such as garlic, onions, soy, coconut, eggs and vinegar.

Sugar

If you want to visibly improve the overall appearance of your skin opt to minimise your sugar intake. This will reduce both inflammation and blotchiness. The negative effects of too much sugar can also be experienced by over consumption of naturally occurring sugars such as fructose in fruit.

Antibiotics and blood pressure medications

While not strictly food, I've put antibiotics and blood pressure medications in this section because they're entering your body and blood stream via the same mechanism.

The impact of antibiotics and blood pressure medications on rosacea is two edged. In the short term, both have been found to either control or exacerbate symptoms. If you are taking either of these medications you need to be aware of the issues and either elect to not take them or seek an alternative drug.

The right antibiotic can successfully control symptoms when you are first diagnosed, especially for papules and/or pimples (pustules), but doesn't seem to have much impact on the overall redness of the skin long term. The wrong antibiotic, however, can lead to an increase in papules and pustules for the duration of the prescription course.

Blood pressure medications have been found to be a source of potential treatment for facial redness and a cause of rosacea flare ups depending on the individual preparations.

What you can do

Stay away from highly processed foods
- Enough said about this already!

Eat Low-histamine foods and DAO promoting foods

● Eat Low-histamine foods and DAO promoting foods such as those listed in Table 3 below - or other foods NOT listed in **Table 1 - Foodstuffs commonly recognised as rosacea triggers.**

Table 3 - Low-histamine foods and DAO promoting foods

Freshly cooked meat (frozen or fresh)	Freshly caught fish	Eggs (including duck eggs)	Gluten-free grains: Rice, Quinoa
Pure peanut butter	Fresh fruits: mango, pear, watermelon, apple, kiwi, cantaloupe, grapes	Fresh vegetables (except tomatoes, spinach, avocado (unless just ripe) and eggplant	Dairy substitutes: coconut milk, rice milk, hemp milk, almond milk
Nuts & seeds: raw cashews, macadamias, hemp seeds	Cooking oils : olive oil, coconut oil, macadamia oil	Leafy herbs	Herbal teas

The key with all these foods is freshness.

Avoid spicy food

● If you go to a restaurant where the food has a tendency to be spicy, order less spicy dishes from the menu.

My experience with certain foods is that, while I don't have a specific flare up at the time, I can find the next morning that my skin has a higher degree of redness. Foods that fall into this category are spicy foods (such as curries) and alcohol.

Avoid multi-tasking while eating

Give eating some priority and singularity in your life

● Avoid eating on the run.

- Avoid the habit of distracted eating while standing, reading or monitoring mobile devices.

Avoid eating too fast

Our busy lifestyles make this one a tough call, but slowing down your eating and savouring your food doesn't take that much longer than you think.

The impact of eating too fast is:

- Increased tendency to overeat because you're not as closely aware of when you're full.
- Increased likelihood you're putting a greater stress on your digestive system by not chewing your food sufficiently.

Try chewing each mouthful at least 10 times as a starting point.

Avoid food/drink that is overly temperature hot, let your food cool down
- Don't gulp down that hot cup of coffee - savour it instead.

Stay hydrated and drink plenty of fluids
- This will also help you to stay cool and will be highly beneficial for the appearance of your skin.

Reduce the amount of dairy products you eat
- An excess of dairy products can lead to greater skin sensitivity in some individuals. [xxi]

Stay vigilant and don't get too casual about the food you eat
- Rosacea is a lifelong condition that never goes away. Don't be tempted to stray too long from your good eating habits.

Introduce natural supplements to your diet
- **Grape seed oil** - has been shown to have a positive impact on reducing inflammation, swelling and vein weakness; it's also an antioxidant. Grapes have been considered to have

medicinal properties for thousands of years. Grape seed oil can either be applied directly to the skin (as an oil or cream), or taken as a supplement in tablet, capsule or liquid forms. My recommendation would be to take it as a supplement for the greatest benefit.

- **Flaxseed oil** - Cold pressed flaxseed oil also reduces redness and inflammation. You can buy the oil in capsule form.

- **Coconut oil** - reduces the appearance of redness when taken internally or applied directly to the skin as a moisturiser.

- **DAO (Diamine Oxidase)** - reduces rosacea symptoms by improving the body's ability to process histamines. This enzyme is available as a supplement in a number of brands.

- **Vitamin B** – ensure you obtain a good supply of B group vitamins either through your food or via a good supplement.

- **Apple cider vinegar** - has been used with great effect to improve the functioning of your stomach and gut. Take a desert spoonful straight up once a day.

Try any of these supplements for approximately 1-2 months. If they don't appear beneficial discontinue them. Then monitor what happens. You may only appreciate the benefits of a supplement once you have stopped taking it. That was my experience with Grape seed oil.

Products/Chemicals applied to the skin or hair
Sheer volume of products

Even the most innocuous toiletry/cosmetic product may have many chemicals listed on the label. Most of the ingredients you've probably never heard of and will be unable to pronounce. I'm not sure if the extent of this labeling is the result of modern manufacturing methods or if governments are now more stringent about product identification - probably a combination of both.

There's certainly plenty of evidence that toiletries and cosmetics are not often required to undergo the same level of testing that's applied to medicines because they're not internally proscribed. This topic has filled countless books on its own. Unfortunately the general population is a giant laboratory for this testing.[xxii]

In an industrialised country on an average day you could be using many or all of the following products (particularly if you're a woman):

Body-wash, shampoo, conditioners, body-gel, leave in conditioner, hairsprays, haircolour, sunscreen, tints, make-up, powders, blush, under arm deodorants, hand cream, eye cream, night cream, foot cream, pore fillers, foundations, concealers, mascaras, eye shadows, eye-liners, lip gloss, lipstick, lip fillers, make-up removers, toners, moisturisers, perfumes, body sprays, nail polishes, nail polish removers, cuticle removers, etc.

There is almost guaranteed to be at least one rosacea trigger in every product you use. When you add these products together you could be applying potentially hundreds of chemicals to your body each day and receiving a strong dose of certain chemicals because they exist in multiple products.

The trigger impacts of cosmetics are a greater issue for women than men but the issue applies to everyone. Men may be even worse off in some respects, as there is not as much societal pressure on them to attend to their appearance, they are more likely to use poor products that are easily available and cheaply made.

This area is hard to tackle because people tend to be strongly wedded to their beauty routines. It's not realistic to promote a 'back to nature' or 'product burning approach' because it's generally impractical for most people. We all have to make our way in the real world and need a workable solution.

Below are some points for navigation:

Products to watch out for or avoid

Products that fall into the following categories should be used sparingly or avoided completely.

Alcohol based

Alcohol is used in cosmetics for its blending and emollient properties. Products that are alcohol based are harsh and drying on your skin. This includes perfumes, toners, witch hazel, hairspray and other hair care products.

Highly scented

Products that are scented can be irritating because they contain both an aromatic (providing the scent) and an alcohol component. The aromatic component is diluted into the alcohol and both are irritants to your skin. Be careful generally with any products that are strongly scented, particularly if you apply them around your face and neck area. Also watch out for scented hand creams as most people have a tendency to touch their face frequently.

Anti-ageing products

Anti-ageing products tend to contain more chemicals than other creams and cosmetics. They can also contain specific abrasive ingredients to create the illusion of smoothness, glow and youth. What they are really providing is an expensive exfoliate or facial scrub which can be too harsh for your skin.

When you see the word anti-aging on a label think: anti-aging = more chemicals + potentially some abrasive qualities.

Propellants

Products that are propellant based such as hairsprays, perfumes, deodorants and dry shampoo etc. need to be applied carefully. In some cases these products have both an alcohol and a propellant base. The key problem is that when you apply these products to different parts of your body you have less control over where they land. Airborne droplets move about freely getting onto your face and other surfaces causing irritation.

Cortisone or steroid medications

Cortisone or steroid medications when applied directly to your face may cause no initial problems but prolonged usage may lead to rosacea flare-ups. [xxiii]

Oils

The following oils sound "natural" but should be avoided because they are too harsh for your skin - especially the skin on your face:

- Peppermint oil
- Eucalyptus oil
- Clove oil
- Menthol oil

Hair care

Hair care products are a source of considerable chemical exposure, particularly if you have chemically treated hair (coloured, permed etc.) and are using additional products to maintain your look. The problem with hair care products is that they don't just stay in your hair. When you wash your hair in the shower the products wash off over your body, get onto your hands and can irritate the skin around your face and neck. I have even read that hair care products can be responsible for conditions such as Athletes Foot[xxiv] because you're standing in the run off shower water when you wash these products out of your hair.

What you can do

Reduce the number of products or brands

- Take an inventory of your bathroom cupboards and makeup bags to start assessing whether you need to be using quite so many products on your skin and hair. The fewer products you use the better, but at the very least try consolidating brands. The amount of chemicals and the techniques manufacturers use to make their products will be similar for all the products across the same brand because they will be made to a price point.

- Try to use the least adulterated products you can find to reduce your chemical exposure.

Read product labels
- Unfortunately even products from heath food stores and products labeled 'organic' can still contain a large number of chemicals. The best advice is to read the label carefully and monitor your use strictly.

Reduce quantities
- Less is more. If you have a tendency to be heavy handed in the way you apply products you may want to start using smaller quantities of some of them to lessen your exposure.

Reduce experimentation
- Cosmetics and toiletries are an area where you want to keep experimentation to an absolute minimum. It can be challenging to resist the power of advertising, but when you settle on products that work don't be tempted to experiment or switch indiscriminately.

Avoid touching your face
- Wash your hands frequently and train yourself out of the habit of touching your face except for the purposes of cleansing and applying makeup. Depending on the order of your beauty routine, this will avoid situations where a product you have just used on your hair gets wiped on your face inadvertently.

- Be careful with highly scented hand creams for the same reason.

- Adopt a gentle cleansing routine and avoid facials, dermabrasion, chemical peels and any other additional "massaging" of the sensitive skin on your face.

Get your hair washed at a salon

- Get your hair washed at a salon or separately to your shower. This is challenging for the average busy person but is an option to consider; even as a temporary solution.

Control the use of propellants

- If you use hairspray try spraying into the cupped palm of your hand and then running it through your hair. Another alternative is to spray outside or somewhere else that is well ventilated. Make sure you wash your hands afterwards.

- The main objective is to keep these products away from your face. If there is a form of the product that doesn't come in an aerosol or propellant I would strongly advise using that form. Otherwise be careful to cover both your face and neck area when you apply these.

Restrict the use of perfume

- If you like to use perfume or aftershave experiment with not applying them on your body any higher than the chest. See if this approach works for you rather than giving them up altogether. You may find that keeping these products away from your face and from behind the ears and neck area will make all the difference.

Avoid the use of toners

- Avoid using alcohol based toners or any toners at all if possible. It's not factual information that using toners to "closes your pores" maintains clearer skin by preventing pimples and blackheads.[xxv] The pores of your skin may increase in size as you age and there really isn't very much you can do about this.[xxvi]

Be vigilant about all forms of chemical contact with your skin

- Change your pillowcase more frequently as chemicals used in cleaning your hair may be rubbing against your face as you sleep. You may want to try using a silk pillowcase, as these are very gentle on your skin particularly if you are a restless sleeper.

● Items of jewelry worn around the neck may pick up chemicals, dirt, oil and shed skin cells that become irritants when worn close to the skin. Ensure you clean these items on a regular basis with nothing harsher than mild soapy water.

● Use a separate towel to dry your hair to reduce chemicals being transferred to your skin.

● Use cleaners and washing detergents with fewer chemicals to reduce the chemical exposure to your skin via your clothes.

Colour tip
● Be cautious with the use of colour. Red tones in both hair colouring and clothing will bring out the redness in your face, so avoid these.

Recommended products

Products for sensitive skin

Most cosmetic brands include a line of products for sensitive skin. These types of products contain fewer chemicals and are usually unscented.

Large brands

The larger cosmetic brands perform a significant amount of hypoallergenic testing on their products that is not always promoted on the packaging. For these companies it's about increasing market share, but this can work in your favour as their products tend to be low in allergens. They are also widely available and reasonably competitive in cost. Avoid getting caught up using brands that are specific, expensive and hard to obtain unless they are really worth your while. Once you find a good brand, stick with it.

Recommended large brands

Neutrogena™, Nivea™, Olay™, Revlon™

Natural alternatives

Rosehip oil and coconut oil
Both can be applied to the skin as soothing moisturisers.

Your mind and lifestyle factors
The Mind / Body connection

Nature AND nurture tend to be factors when assessing illnesses caused by a disruption to the body's defense mechanisms. While there's been limited research done on the link between rosacea and personality a number of findings can be presented:

- 91% of people report that the first onset of rosacea is typically preceded by a traumatic episode or a period of intense stress[xxvii] (mentioned previously in relation to pregnancy and menopause).
- Rosacea sufferers have a higher incidence of depression.[xxviii]
- Rosacea sufferers rated lower on scores of verbal aggression when compared to other people in an office study.[xxix]
- Only 52% of rosacea sufferers can trace a clear genetic link to another family member who also has the condition. [xxx]

These findings both shed light on what else may be going in a person's life to create a primed environment for rosacea to emerge and add more complexity into the mix, further confusing the identification of cause and effect factors.

Stereotyping a rosacea personality type is risky, but it would be fair to say there do seem to be strong personality traits that may indicate a susceptibility to rosacea:

- High tendency to anxiety and stress
- Lack of assertiveness skills or clear boundaries with others
- Highly sensitive and/or introverted
- Perfectionist tendencies
- Certain rigidity of outlook and unwillingness to embrace change
- High tendency to hold on to the past

These personality traits may have been a feature of a person's whole life or they may have developed more recently in response to current circumstances.

If a number of these traits apply you may want to consider what else is going on in your life right now that could be exacerbating your rosacea

Social factors and perceptions

A recent interesting study was conducted which highlighted people's negative perception of rosacea symptoms.[xxxi] The study was established to gauge social reactions to people who have clear versus less clear complexions. People who exhibited rosacea symptoms were viewed as less confident and more shy, nervous and stressed. They were also more likely to be perceived as unhealthy in some way. Rosacea sufferers themselves, in social situations, tended to be self-conscious and worried about the redness of their skin and their appearance over other factors. This preoccupation undermined their general sense of enjoyment in social settings.

There have been plenty of studies done about the social feedback loops that operate between individuals. This feedback system affects the way people behave, are perceived and the manner in which others respond to them.[xxxii] This applies particularly to attributes such as attractiveness, race, gender etc. These perceptions and responses shape people powerfully over a lifetime. Consequently the negative social impacts of rosacea cannot be underestimated, particularly in interactions with the opposite sex. The amount of confidence a person displays, the extent to which they see themselves as worthy of acceptance and their capacity to engage unselfconsciously in social activities can be undermined by excessive worry about the appearance of their rosacea symptoms. This becomes a 'chicken and egg' scenario.

Emotional anxiety – Stress

If you experience high levels of stress and anxiety your rosacea is not a beneficial response to the situation because it's like having a sign over your head that screams to the world "I'm feeling stressed!"

There's been an enormous amount written about the "fight or flight" syndrome and the extent to which modern living can over stimulate these protective responses. It would be valuable to learn some relaxation techniques to reduce your anxiety and stress response to the types of situations you regularly encounter.

Relaxation techniques

Breathing

When you're feeling under stress your body tenses and your breathing often becomes quite shallow. Highly anxious individuals experience shallow breathing most of the time. The subsequent effect is that carbon dioxide stays in your system for longer.[xxxiii] People vary in the extent to which this carbon dioxide build affects them. Some people become significantly affected and anxious at lower levels while for others the amount has to get quite significant before they are conscious of discomfort.

Concentrating on your breathing is probably the most primal relaxation technique; something that all great teachers and mystics seem to come back to repeatedly. The idea that breath is life is a powerful one. If you stop breathing it's 'game over' pretty quickly - way faster than being without water or food. If you can develop the habit of more conscious breathing you will be able to better overcome your reflexive stress responses.

Below are two techniques which can be practiced consciously anywhere to slow your breathing down. Both these techniques will distract you from your anxieties by distracting you to concentrate on your breathing. They can be used in situations where you feel your stress levels rising and need a quick method to calm yourself. You might be waiting for a job interview, a date or in any other situation where you can feel yourself flushing and you're becoming stressed you won't be looking your best at the critical moment.

Simple breathing technique - One

A technique to slow down your breathing while counting your inhale and exhale breaths.

- Breath in for the count of 5
- Hold your breath for the count of 5
- Breath out for the count of 5
- REPEAT the cycle 5 times

Simple breathing technique - Two

Variation on technique one.

- Place your tongue on the small ridge between the top of your first teeth and the roof of your mouth
- Breath in through your mouth for the count of 3
- Hold your breath for a few counts
- Breath out through your nose for the count of 5

REPEAT 3-4 times and you will feel considerably more relaxed.

The trick to this technique is that you must keep your tongue in the one place and concentrate on your count for of the duration of your breathing.

Meditation

Meditation is another conscious relaxation practice that can be extremely effective and doesn't need to be something you do for hours a day sitting cross-legged on a mat. Meditation can be done for as little as five to ten minutes a day. The key is to do a small amount regularly as part of your daily routine. Ten minutes done every day will be of far greater benefit than two hours done once a week.

Find somewhere private and quiet where you won't be disturbed. Sitting cross-legged on a floor, couch or bed is great but if you're not able to do that just relax in a chair or lie on the floor. The main thing is to get into a habit.

Sit comfortably, set a timer for five to ten minutes (mobile phone alarms are great for this and also extremely portable). Close your eyes and try to empty your thoughts. At first this will be hard and you might race through your "To Do" lists and all the things on your mind. But don't worry; just gently try to bring your mind back to not thinking about much at all. Concentrate on your breathing, relax your body, feel your senses, experience the moment. Breath deeply into your body using your diaphragm.

After doing this practice every day you will start to feel some changes. You will feel more grounded and less stressed in social situations and will experience a lot less worry overall. Most importantly, you will find it easier to slip into a relaxed state even when not meditating, because you have been in the habit of experiencing relaxation more regularly.

Guided meditation

Some people are more comfortable with a guided meditation. This is a short meditation where you listen to a recording of someone guiding you through relaxation steps. The effectiveness of prerecorded meditations may vary. I personally am not a fan, preferring to experience silence. Your level of comfort with this approach will depend largely on how well you relate to the voice of the person on the recording. You'll have to decide for yourself whether this type of meditation works for you. The last thing you want is to listen to an irritating voice, it will just be annoying and the very opposite of relaxing!

Sleeping and napping

Your body has amazing powers of self-repair and rejuvenation, but it needs adequate rest to carry out these processes. Many view a regular good night's sleep as a secret weapon. All those adages about eating properly, exercising regularly and getting plenty of rest are truer now more than ever in our lives. Your body will benefit and your rosacea will significantly improve with adequate rest.

People vary in the amount of sleep they need. Humans got considerably more sleep in an earlier age before the invention of the electric light bulb.[xxxiv] If you are chronically tired, irritable, depressed, have low sex drive, weight issues, or are overly emotional or angry - these are all potential signs you could be lacking sleep. Ironically, one of the key signs you're sleep deprived is poor judgment about your sleep patterns and the effect it's having on your physical and mental well-being! Sleep is not a waste of time; it's a productivity tool.

Start by aiming for eight hours a night and assess from there.

Assertiveness and self-awareness

If you're someone who's not particularly assertive this can be another source of stress and anxiety further contributing to your rosacea symptoms. The distinction between assertion and aggression is often not well understood. Assertiveness is about stating your rights and establishing reasonable boundaries with other people; aggression is about domination. Usually people who are weak in assertiveness skills have not seen this skill well demonstrated in their family environment. Vague boundaries with other people can leave you floundering and anxious, but it's a skill that can be developed through practice. Improved assertiveness will enable you to negotiate your needs respectfully and clearly in social situations and with family members.

Counselling

It may be valuable to talk to a counselor or therapist while you're gaining control over your rosacea. A trained professional can offer insights into your behaviour and ensure a level of discretion. A therapist will allow you to get some focused "me" time that doesn't put pressure on you to reciprocate as you would be expected to do with a friend.

If you are someone who's potentially isolated and tends to hold the world at arms' length, creating the opportunity to talk freely about your emotions in a safe environment may be the problem you need to address.

Something about avoidance

There's a famous statistic that people are more fearful of dying than speaking in public.[xxxv] If you're like most people you've probably done your best to avoid situations where you're required to speak or be the center of attention. This avoidance tendency can become pronounced for rosacea sufferers who live in dread of a public red-faced display.

Travelling under the radar or shuffling to the back of the crowd may seem like the best survival strategy, but you're actually doing yourself a disservice. The more you try to avoid these situations, the worse they become in your mind and in reality. Avoidance isn't really an effective solution; it's the path of least resistance

A far better strategy is to proactively seek out these types of situations (public speaking, job interviews, first dates, meetings at work, speeches etc.) and become desensitised to them through more frequent exposure. When you develop the skills to perform well at these moments and practice regular relaxation techniques you should be able to rise to these occasions with style.

What you can do

Visualisation

- Get a flattering photo of yourself with clear skin or of you looking your best and smiling (maybe in a social situation). Put this photo where you can refer to it every day or whenever you want. The photo will be a powerful form of visualisation to get you focusing on your goal and not just your symptoms.

Relaxation and rest

- Practice relaxation techniques such as meditation to assist you to deal with anxious situations.

- Get plenty of sleep. This will allow your body to fully repair and regenerate itself. It will also help you to manage your anxiety symptoms.

Seek professional help

- Investigate other programs available such as hypnotherapy and/or Cognitive Behavioural Therapy (CBT). The latter will be particularly helpful if you feel caught in a loop and have developed a strong degree of social anxiety about your condition.

- Develop your assertiveness skills.

Join a support group

- Join an online rosacea support group or start a group locally.

Review your lifestyle

- Assess some of your friendships and your lifestyle. Unhealthy choices around food and drink can be heavily influenced by your peer group, which may be having an impact on your capacity to make changes.

- Review your close relationships or lack of them.

- Think about the type of recreation activities you do.

- Ask yourself whether you are a person who is resistant to change.

Review your environment
- Assess your chosen profession or work environment, it could be a source of excessive stress.

- Assess the type of buildings you live and work in.

Ease up on yourself
- Be kinder to yourself when you're having a particularly bad red-faced day or incident - you are getting this under control.

Chapter 3 - Treating Your Rosacea

Managing Rosacea in a social context

I've now reached the stage where my rosacea is relatively under control and I don't fear certain foods if they are served up to me in somebody's home.

When I want to avoid a certain food I just use the phrase: "I don't eat/drink x; it doesn't agree with me", and leave it at that. I do this all the time with beer. People tend not to delve further as many people have issues with foods they either don't like or which don't agree with them.

Where you may strike problems is when you *start* moderating your diet. The people who prepare your meals or dine with you on a regular basis may see these changes as a form of rejection, particularly if you are rejecting traditional or ethnic cuisine.

Using a counsellor or therapist may be a good strategy to support you while navigating new forms of negotiation with others. At this stage don't think you have to talk about your rosacea in the presence of people you don't know well. You are not your condition - it doesn't define you. You don't have to take on the role of proselytiser if that's not comfortable to you.

Relaxation and meditation techniques will assist you to push through social situations when you have symptoms. Keep your red face in perspective. You are worthy of acceptance and the more quickly you can move your mind on from your condition the lesser the symptoms will be. A more relaxed mindset will help you to manage social situations because you will not be as anxious. Remember everyone else is way more focused on themselves than they are focused on you.

On a practical front

When you're socialising with people with whom you're "thermally incompatible" it can be a source of tension, but it's important to appreciate that your rights as not lesser to theirs. Unless they are infants! By thermally incompatible I mean people who are either much more or much less sensitive to heat or cold then yourself. Or as is often the case, people who don't like to 'rug up' and would prefer to manage their comfort by turning the heating up or down. This can be difficult at times, but compromises can be negotiated in most situations.

If you are at a venue be conscious of seat positioning near heating sources in rooms (like open fires) and don't be afraid to be assertive if you need the heat turned down or the air conditioning turned on. Don't be backward about making the same requests when travelling in taxis either. Simply state your needs clearly.

Outdoor gas heaters positioned on high stands can be a trap. These radiate heat straight down onto your head and face, which can be extremely uncomfortable. In most situations you can elect to sit somewhere else at the table or ask the venue staff to turn the heaters down or off.

The more proactive you are and the more in advance conversations you can have the better. If you are going out it may be useful to visit the place beforehand or get some intelligence from someone who is familiar with the venue. If you're invited to someone's house for a meal don't wait until the meal is being served to mention you have a problem with the food. Tell the host at the point of invitation. Similarly if you are changing the foods that you eat at home discuss these changes before meals are planned and shopping is done rather than at the point where the meal is being prepared or placed in front of you. This behaviour can be interpreted as rude when people have gone to some effort to prepare a meal and is almost guaranteed to cause an awkward situation.

Some useful phrases

Here are some useful phrases to help you navigate your way socially:

- "I don't eat/drink x; it doesn't agree with me" - to avoid consuming a trigger food.

- "It was beautiful and I would love some more but I'm really full". - When you have consumed a trigger food and don't want any more.

- "I feel uncomfortably warm. Is it possible to turn down the heating". - When you are negotiating thermal rights with others.

- "How can we both be comfortable with this temperature/situation". - When you are negotiating thermal rights with others.

- "I'm not going to be able to sit here, it's too warm, can I swap with you". - When you are negotiating seating further away from a heating source

- "I feel very warm here, is it possible to turn down the heating or switch to another table". - When you are dealing with restaurant or venue staff.

- "Thank you for the invitation. I eat almost anything but I do have a problem with x or y they don't agree with me. I hope that's not a problem". - Before you go to someone's house for a meal to ensure that the meal does not contain dominant triggers

- "I've been diagnosed with a condition called rosacea. As part of the treatment I've had to modify my eating habits. I'm no longer able to eat x and y". - When dealing with change and reactions from others around food and meals.

- "I'm letting you know that as part of identifying my rosacea triggers I am going to stop eating x for a while". - When dealing with change and reactions from others around food and meals.

Setting up a Daily Trigger Diary

Set up a mechanism that works best for you with your trigger diary. Use paper, electronic or just keep track of everything in a journal. You'll also find some excellent apps in iTunes and Google Play. Keep it simple and easy to refer back to.

Data to collect

- Date
- Time of Day
- What else might have been going on - are you at work, weekend, holiday etc.
- Did you eat or try something new - include any new foods eaten, beverages consumed, new or existing toiletry/cosmetic products tried.
- Mention if you skip meals or are particularly dehydrated for some reason.
- Have you been in particularly stressful situations such as a high profile meeting or a meal in a restaurant with people you don't know very well.

Once you start your diary and begin analysing the data you'll begin to see patterns in your regular behaviour. The things you do frequently will become particularly obvious. For example, how often you eat certain foods, experience stress or use certain products etc., which may be more often than you realise. When you start eliminating items from your diet or from your daily beauty routine you will find the remaining triggers much easier to identify because there will be progressively fewer of them to track.

Table 4 - Diary sample

Date	Time	Observation	Notes

Table 5 - Diary sample - filled in

Date	Time	Observation	Notes
Mon day 1/6	8:45am	Arrived at work, flushed as I entered the building. Cold morning Temperature 5°C (41°F)	Need to protect my face better in the cold. Maybe walk slower.
" "	10:30am	Went out for coffee with Melissa. Still cold got flushed entering the coffee place and re-entering our building	Felt anxious thinking about flushing again.
" "	12:30pm	Ate lunch at my desk, didn't leave the building but flushed. Had a chicken pasta dish with cheese reheated?	Not caused by cold but potentially chicken, cheese, and food temperature?
" "	5:30pm	Left work, air temperature warmer no flushing on train	

Date	Time	Observation	Notes
		trip home.	
" "	7:00pm	Dinner - Steak and vegetables	No flushing, felt relaxed
" "	10:30pm	Showered for bed - cleansed off make up, put long lasting conditioner in hair	Skin felt burning, could be a few things here - heat of the shower, face cleansing products or routine, conditioner?
Tues day 2/6	6:30am	Got up, face a bit blotchy	bedding too warm? conditioner? less likely dinner
" "	8:50am	Arrived at work, not flushing when entering building - outside temperature warmer 17°C (62.8°F)	:-)
" "	10:00am	Important team meeting to chair got very flushed in the room	The room was too small for the number of people and hot. I felt anxious and tense.
" "	12:40pm	Lunch - dived out and got a sandwich (Cheese and lettuce) no flushing	Temperature warm 20°C (68°F)

Date	Time	Observation	Notes
" "	5:15pm	Left work and stopped for a quick drink with Carole - 1 glass of champagne	No flushing, felt relaxed
" "	7:00pm	Dinner at home - zucchini pasta bake and salad	No flushing
	11:00pm	Showered for bed, cleansed off make up	Skin felt burning - no conditioner but shower? skin cleansing?

This completed sample diary has examples of all the things you need be thinking about: environment, food, products and state of mind. This sample shows our person at the beginning of the process of analysing their triggers. In some cases there are multiple items that *may* be triggers and need to be broken down further.

From just a couple of day's worth of diary you can see some patterns emerging:

Cold weather
- Our person, let's call them Jenny, clearly has a problem with cold outside temperatures and transitioning between hot and cold environments. You see this when she entered her work place on the first day and also went in and out mid-morning for a coffee when it was still relatively cold. But she didn't have the same issue the next morning when the air temperature was warmer.

TO THINK ABOUT: Protecting her skin more when outside, walking more slowly, being extra careful on cold days.

State of mind
- Clearly Jenny's state of mind along with the cold seems to be a factor.

TO THINK ABOUT: Know that cold weather is a factor and as well as protecting her skin, needing to practice relaxation techniques and anticipate a potential problem in these types of climate conditions.

Identification of "no trigger" meals
- The meal eaten on the first night (steak and vegetables) seemed to be ok, caused no flushing this is a good tip. Mental note that this is a meal that could be ordered safely when the Jenny is out in public at a restaurant.

- Lunch and dinner on the second day did not lead to incidents of flushing so that is a good indicator that those are thumbs up 'ok' foods for rosacea.

Cleansing routine needs attention
- Both nights when Jenny finished up her evening routine she had a burning sensation to her face. The heat of the shower and the cleansing routine were common factors to both nights. So these are places to start.
- She woke up with a blotchy face on the second morning and there could be a few indicators here - the pre-bed bathroom routine or the heat of the bed clothes.

TO THINK ABOUT: The issue is mostly likely to be the cleansing routine because that is the part of the pre-bed routine that is most concerned with the face. I would not rule out the other factors but this is where I would start to make a change to the products used, the heaviness of the touch to the face for starters.

Overheated rooms and state of mind

• Jenny reported getting anxious and tense in the team meeting she was chairing. She also made the observation that the room was too small for the number of people.

TO THINK ABOUT: Both these factors were probably in play. Organising for the meeting to be held in a more appropriate room, if possible. Preparation and more practice with chairing would also be a good option.

State of mind and alcohol

• The glass of champagne with the friend after work did not appear to lead to flushing. This is valuable information because if champagne causes a problem on another occasion then it's probably not the champagne but other factors such as state of mind, the company and/or the ambient temperature.

Putting it all together into a program

In the previous sections we've identified the key areas impacting your rosacea:

- Genetics
- Environment
- Foods
- Products applied to skin and hair
- Mind and lifestyle
- Other related disorders and conditions

We've also talked about how your body is not a machine and that people differ as to the relative importance of each trigger. We've also covered how to set up your Daily Trigger Diary.

Here's an approach to treatment that ties it all together.

An approach to treatment

1. **Set up your photo** - Put your photo of yourself looking your best in a prominent place - Visualise.

2. **Familiarise yourself with trigger foods and products** - Become familiar with the foods and types of products I've listed, particularly the foods and products you use on a regular basis.

3. **Commence your Daily Trigger Diary** - Analyse each previous day and each previous week so that you can start to understand your cycles and patterns.

4. **Start assessing your reactions to cosmetics** - If you are someone who uses a number of cosmetic products I would start with the things you are putting on your face directly and then work out from there to other parts of the body. Work from the head down starting with face, neck, head/hair, then hands.

5. **Avoid touching your face unnecessarily** - If you tend to be a someone who fidgets, this will be challenging initially but over time will become second nature.

6. **Protect yourself from the environment** - Environment is probably the biggest challenge because it's usually the trigger factor that's under the least of your control. But what you can do is:
   - Moisturise well
   - Stay hydrated
   - Slow down your transition between hot and cold temperatures
   - Protect the skin on your face with collars, scarves or hoods

7. **Meditation** - Start mediating or practicing another relaxation technique every day.

8. **Start cautious elimination of foods/products** - Based on the patterns you're seeing in your Daily Trigger Diary start cautious elimination of products and/of foods.
   - Start with removing potential trigger foods that you eat frequently.

9. **Relax** - Relax and move at your own pace, it's not a race.

10. **Listen to your body** - Start to become sensitive to changes occurring in your body and how you are feeling over the course of each day. You may have been living with a level of discomfort for some time so need to acclimatise yourself to a new feeling of 'normal'.

11. **Celebrate your wins**
    - My first big win was the removal of Parmesan cheese from my diet. I'm a big pasta lover and was sprinkling Parmesan cheese over my meals almost every day. Hard

cheeses, like Parmesan, are on the list of suspect foods. While I was getting my condition to settle I avoided all hard cheeses completely. Now my skin is under control I'm able to have Parmesan sprinkled on my food with no effect. The psychological boost of this first big win cannot be underestimated. For the first time I felt I would be able to gain control over my condition.

12. **Get support** - Don't go it alone - look for support groups online, talk to your partner, family or others you can trust, consider counseling.

13. **Repeat** - all of the above steps

If you pursue this course of diary, feedback and correction you should be in a greatly improved position with your rosacea within a couple of months and will have established sustainable routines you can take forward.

Key things to remember at this point

Eliminate one thing at a time and make an assessment

Be scientific and eliminate one thing at a time. I can't stress the importance of this enough. This approach will take you less time in the long run and enable you to exert greater control over your condition sooner. It will also avoid the potential for unnecessary elimination of foods or chemicals that are not the problem.

It's tempting to start cutting out and changing many things at once because you're overwhelmed with new information and want to see fast results. But resist this temptation, as it will only cause confusion. If it helps, potentially alter only one item in each category at a time: one skincare product and one food, for example.

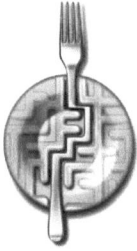

Examine EVERYTHING

This includes products and foods you may have been using / consuming for a very long time and that you love and may not want to relinquish. Also be conscious of beverages, it can be easy to overlook their impact and not take them as seriously as solid food. In my case, two of my triggers were beer and diet coke.

Resist too much experimentation

At least until you gain a better sense of control over your condition management. One of the other sneaky aspects of rosacea is that you may try something new like a cosmetic on your skin and the product may be fine for a number of days. You may be able to use a new cosmetic for even as long as two weeks before you get a flare up that's in direct response to the new product, by this time you've completely forgotten your experiment. You may think this new product is just awesome and through coincidence mistakenly attribute a flare up to some other cause i.e. something you may have just eaten, sending you down a dead end.

Focus on yourself

Use this period to focus on yourself and potentially to take some time out. You may also find it valuable to keep a journal of your thoughts and feelings. Use it to chart your journey with rosacea so you can celebrate the wins and appreciate just how far you've come. It will also be another potential source for trigger patterns.

A word of caution

You'll reach a point where your symptom management system becomes so refined you no longer have rosacea at the forefront of your mind anymore. This is your ultimate goal, but remember rosacea never completely goes away.

There will be occasions when you are travelling, under stress or just generally out of your normal routine when you'll find yourself vulnerable to forgetting that your rosacea is something you still have to actively manage. Under these circumstances you'll quickly find that if you become too casual your symptoms will return. For example you may be able to have a celebratory beer at the end of the working week with no real affect. But if you're on holiday and find yourself having a couple of glasses of beer every afternoon then your system will quickly flare up and your symptoms will return.

Phases of treatment

You'll notice two distinct phases of your treatment: **Identification** and **Maintenance**

In the **Identification** phase you'll isolate your specific triggers and eliminate them until you skin calms down. You'll then move into the **Maintenance** phase where you'll have your rosacea largely under control apart from the odd flare up.

In the **Maintenanc***e* phase you'll be able to reintroduce foods you previously eliminated with little or no reaction. This can be enormously helpful in social situations when you are inadvertently served up trigger food. If you've been practicing your relaxation techniques regularly your sense of control over your rosacea will contribute to a heightened sense of wellbeing.

Once you reach the routine level of the **Maintenance** phase you can then make an assessment as to whether you want to refine your systems further or already have the situation under sufficient control. This will depend on the outcome you want to pursue.

Costs $$$

Getting control of your rosacea can be expensive of your time as well as your money. This can be the cause of additional stress as you spend money visiting doctors, trying supplements, buying books, throwing out cosmetics, buying new products, paying for prescription medication, buying additional clothing etc.

You don't have to do everything at once. To help maximise your efforts I would focus on the following priority order:

- Doctors / Specialists - this shouldn't involve more than a couple of appointments (if it involves more, I would be concerned about the quality of the specialist).
- Food - changes to diet
- Relaxation techniques
- Cosmetics
- Changes to clothing

You don't need to break the bank to improve your situation.

Good luck! You're on your way!

Disclaimer

The obligatory part -

This book is intended to increase your knowledge about your condition and provide you with further information. I'm not a medical person and this book is not intended to be a substitute for the medical advice of a qualified medical practitioner. The reader should regularly consult a qualified medical practitioner in matters relating to his/her health and particularly with respect to any symptoms that may require diagnosis or medical attention. Reference to specific brands and products do not exclude the use of other brands and products omitted. Brand names, logos and trademarks used herein remain the property of their respective owners.

About the author

I'm a fellow rosacea sufferer and have been diagnosed for about 15 years. Today, apart from a few telltale moments, very few people are able to pick that I have rosacea and I frequently get comments about my beautiful skin. I went on quite a roller coaster with this condition myself so know what you're grappling with.

I fully understand the impact rosacea is having on your life and how it undermines your confidence. I've written this book as a friend to show you there is a way forward and you can beat this.

I had always been someone who blushed easily, particularly in social situations and the skin around my neck often had a blotchy appearance. As I was approaching my forties I started to notice the redness on my cheeks had became almost permanent. I tried various products to hide this, but it wasn't until I was away on holidays one year that I realised I had a major problem and my face looked far worse than I thought. I looked at my skin by a particularly unflattering light in the bathroom mirror and saw I had a number of what I thought were pimples and the underlying redness of my face had spread over a much larger area.

I subsequently stumbled across the word 'rosacea' one day in a magazine. I investigated further and was able to connect rosacea to my symptoms - a Eureka moment!

I finally had a condition with a name I could work with.

When I turned forty my father put together a photo album of myself and different members of our family. My paternal grandmother had a sister and two brothers. There were a couple of photos of the group of siblings from different points in their lives and there, in a photo of the older group, were the telltale signs of rosacea on the face of my great uncle. There the family genetic basis, further proof I wasn't adopted (ha ha!).

Chloe Hill can be contacted via her publisher at info@stivesmedia.com.au

Author thanks

Books don't write themselves that is the author's role. But no book is ever completely a solo production. Many people have supported the writing of this book but I would like to make particular mention of the following:

I would like to thank my husband and fellow author Alan - whose love, encouragement and technical advice was the make or break for this project.

For all their moral support throughout this project. You always believed in me:
Melissa, Erika, Jean, Suzanne, Sarah and Jane.

For her expert health advice I would like to thank:
Vesna.

All errors and missteps are wholly my own :-(:)

Further references

Books

Chase, Deborah **The New Medically-Based No-Nonsense Beauty Book**, Holt and Co, 1992.

Hay, Louise L. **You can heal your life** Specialist Publications, 1984.
Kind of 'The Bible' on mind / body medicine.

Holbrook, Georgie **Joy-full holistic remedies: How to experience your natural ability to heal** Joy-Full Publishing Company, 1999
One of the most impactive books I've read in this area. Georgie Holbroke went on a significant journey to heal some painful issues in her own life and consequently her rosacea. I can really recommend this book because it is from the trenches and is Georgie telling her own story about getting on top of rosacea.

Holiday, Ryan **The Obstacle is the way : the timeless art of turning trials into triumphs** Portfolio, 2014
A valuable and inspirational book and pushing through adversity and using obstacles in your life to your advantage.

Maas, James **Power sleep**, William Morrow, 1998.

Molloy, Hugh & Egger, Gary **Skin fitness: safe and healthy skin care**, Allen & Unwin, 2008
A great all round discussion about keeping your skin healthy and what not to do.

Nase, Geoffrey Dr. **Beating Rosacea: vascular, ocular & acne forms - a must have guide to understanding & treating rosacea** Nase Publications 2001
Another seminal work on rosacea written by a medical doctor about his own research, analysis and management of the condition.

Internet resources

The Internet will assist you with finding out more about your condition and connecting with other rosacea sufferers from around the world. To list a few of the great websites and support groups here:

• A comprehensive online medical resource site
Medicine.net.com
http://www.medicinenet.com/rosacea/page7.htm

• Home of the National Rosacea Society of America
rosacea.org

• A good online rosacea forum
rosaceagroup.org

Dermatologists

Your doctor will be able to refer you to a dermatologist. You may be able to see a specialist directly but this may interfere with the terms of your medical claims and rebates. Check first with your health insurance fund.

Guided meditation resources

iTunes store

Google Play

Both of these sites will also be sources for trigger diary apps.

■ ■ ■

About the publisher

St Ives Media is a publishing house based in Melbourne, Australia. Check out our range of titles at stivesmedia.com.au

If you would like further information please contact us on: info@stivesmedia.com.au

Notes

[i] American Heritage® Dictionary of the English Language, Fifth Edition. Copyright © 2011 by Houghton Mifflin Harcourt Publishing Company. Published by Houghton Mifflin Harcourt Publishing Company.

[ii] businesswire.com (April 22 2014) 'New survey finds people with rosacea are more likely to be judged negatively upon first impression than people with clear skin' . Retrieved August 18 2015.

[iii] medicinenet.com - Retrieved August 18 2015.

[iv] medicinenet.com - Retrieved August 18 2015.

[v] rosacea.org National Rosacea Society of America - Retrieved April 21 2015

[vi] Zouboulis, Christos, Katsambas, Andreas, Albert M. Kligman (ed.) Pathogenesis and treatment of acne rosacea. Springer 28 July 2014 p. 670.

[vii] 'Rosacea inflammation and aging : the inefficiency of stress' by Ray Peat raypeat.com Retrieved August 7 2015.

[viii] Blount, B. Wayne, Pelletier Allen L. 'Rosacea a common, yet commonly overlooked condition'. www.aafp.org › Journals › afp › Vol. 66/No. 3 (August 1, 2002)

[ix] 'The most overlooked rosacea treatment: targeting damaged lymphatic vessels' by Dr Geoffrey Nase (September 3 2014) drones.drnase.com retrieved August 20 2015.

[x] 'How to balance stomach acid and improve acne and rosacea fast!' by Christa Orecchio n.d. thewholejourney.com retrieved August 20 2015.

[xi] Enders, Giulia Gut : the inside story of our bodies most underrated organ Scribe Publications, 2015.

xii rosacea.org National Rosacea Society of America - Retrieved April 21 2015

xiii Peat, Ray "Rosacea, inflammation and aging : The inefficiency of stress" retrieved August 9 2015 from raypeat.com

xiv 'Rosacea and personality' by Erik Karlsson, Mats Berg and Bengt B. Arnetz in Acta Derm Venreol 84, August 2003.

xv Peat, Ray "Rosacea, inflammation and aging : The inefficiency of stress" retrieved August 9 2015 from raypeat.com

xvi Peat, Ray "Rosacea, inflammation and aging : The inefficiency of stress" retrieved August 9 2015 from raypeat.com

xvii 'Freshness counts ; histamine intolerance' by Georgia Ede M.D. diagnosisdiet.com n.d. retrieved May 20 2015.

xviii 'Food sources of nitrates and nitrites: the physiologic context for potential health benefits' by Norman G. Hord, Yaoping Tang and Nathan S. Bryan. American Journal of Clinical Nutrition Vol 90. no 1 May 2009.

xix L'hirondel, Jean Nitrate and man : Toxic, harmful or beneficial? CABI 2009.

xx 'Food sources of nitrates and nitrites: the physiologic context for potential health benefits' by Norman G. Hord, Yaoping Tang and Nathan S. Bryan. American Journal of Clinical Nutrition Vol 90. no 1 May 2009.

xxi 'Dairy intolerance: Lactose intolerance, Casein allergy' December 11 2013 http://www.foodintol.com/dairy-intolerance, Retrieved August 201 2015.

xxii Chase, Deborah The New Medically-Based No-Nonsense Beauty Book, Holt and Co, 1992.

xxiii 'Steroid induced rosacea' dermishealth.com retrieved August 22 2015.

[xxiv] Molloy, Hugh & Egger, Gary Skin fitness: safe and healthy skin care, Allen & Unwin, 2008 p. 72.

[xxv] 'Time to bin your toner!' by Natasha Devon, April 29 2013 dailymail.co.uk Retrieved August 22 2015.

[xxvi] "10 myths & misconceptions about skincare' by Carolyn Ash. carolynash.com n.d. Retrieved August 22 2015

[xxvii] 'Rosacea and personality' by Erik Karlsson, Mats Berg and Bengt B. Arnetz in Acta Derm Venreol 84, August 2003.

[xxviii] Peat, Ray "Rosacea, inflammation and aging : The inefficiency of stress" retrieved August 9 2015 from raypeat.com

[xxix] 'Rosacea and personality' by Erik Karlsson, Mats Berg and Bengt B. Arnetz in Acta Derm Venreol 84, August 2003.

[xxx] rosacea.org National Rosacea Society of America - Retrieved April 21 2015

[xxxi] businesswire.com (April 22 2014) 'New survey finds people with rosacea are more likely to be judged negatively upon first impression than people with clear skin' . Retrieved August 18 2015.

[xxxii] 'The Truth about why beautiful people are more successful' by Dario Maestripieri March 8 2012 psychology today.com Retrieved August 22 2015.

[xxxiii] 'New insight into panic attacks: Carbon dioxide is the culprit' by Gowda Shilpa, November 2007 jyi.org Retrieved August 22 2015.

[xxxiv] Maas, James Power sleep , William Morrow, 1998.

[xxxv] 'The Thing we fear more than death' by Glenn Croston, November 29 2012 psychology today.com Retrieved August 22 2015.